Table of Contents

Pancreatitis is an inflammation (swelling) of the pancreas. When the pancreas is inflamed, the powerful digestive enzymes it makes can damage its tissue. The inflamed pancreas can cause release of inflammatory cells and toxins that may harm your lungs, kidneys and heart.

There are two forms of pancreatitis:

Acute pancreatitis is a sudden and short bout of inflammation.

Chronic pancreatitis is ongoing inflammation.

1. Freezer Sweet Potato Waffles (Extra Crispy)

Prep Time: 20 Minutes

Cook Time: 10 Minutes

Servings: 3

Ingredients

- 1 cup sweet potato puree
- ¾ cup milk
- 1 egg
- ¼ cup oil *see note
- ¾ cup flour can use half whole wheat
- ⅓ cup cornmeal
- 2 teaspoons baking powder
- 1 teaspoon salt

Instructions

1. Prepare your sweet potato puree by steaming roughly 2.5 cups of ½ inch sweet potato cubes for 10 minutes or until soft. Mash or blend with a hand mixer until smooth.
2. Combine the sweet potato puree with milk, egg and oil, and mix until completely combined.
3. In a separate bowl, combine the flour, cornmeal, baking powder and salt.
4. Combine the wet and dry ingredients and mix until just combined.
5. Cook on a greased waffle maker (I use spray oil) until cooked through. On my waffle maker, this was 3-4 minutes.
6. Serve immediately or allow to cool completely.
7. Storage
8. To freeze: Wrap in plastic wrap, or in plastic bags. Combine individual portions in a large ziplock freezer bag.
9. To thaw: Place frozen waffles in the toaster, and toast until crisp and heated through

2. Cottage Cheese Pancakes

Prep Time: 15 Minutes

Cook Time: 15 Minutes

Servings: 5

Ingredients

- 1 cup cottage cheese
- 2 eggs
- 2 tablespoons maple syrup
- ½ teaspoon vanilla
- 1 cups white whole wheat flour 125 g; fluffed, spooned & levelled;
- 1 teaspoons baking powder
- ¼ teaspoon salt
- ¼ cup milk optional;

Instructions

1. Mix the wet ingredients– Star by mixing together the wet ingredients: add the cottage cheese, eggs, maple syrup and vanilla. Mix with a spatula until the batter is well combined.

2. Mix in the dry ingredients- Place the flour, baking powder and salt onto the wet mixture. Mix until no pockets of flour remain. At this point, you can assess whether the batter needs milk to thin it out; see the photo above for the desired consistency. If adding milk, start with ¼ cup, then add more as needed.

3. Prepare the pan- Heat a nonstick pan over medium heat for 1-2 minutes. Spray with oil, or grease well with olive or vegetable oil.

4. Cook the pancakes- Measure out ¼ cup portions and place into the greased pan. Pat into a circular shape, then cook for roughly 2 minutes, or until golden. Flip and cook for 1-2 additional minutes. Transfer to a wire rack to rest while you cook the other pancakes.

5. Serve- Serve the pancakes with berries and syrup, or serve with savory ingredients such as bacon and scrambled eggs.

6. Cook the pancakes- Measure out ¼ cup portions and place into the greased pan. Pat into a circular shape, then cook for roughly 2 minutes, or until golden. Flip and cook for 1-2 additional minutes. Transfer to a wire rack to rest while you cook the other pancakes.

7. Serve- Serve the pancakes with berries and syrup, or serve with savory ingredients such as bacon and scrambled eggs.

8. Tips:

9. we've used 2% cottage cheese in this recipe; non-fat cottage cheese should also work fine. Avoid dry curd cottage cheese, which could alter the liquid content of the recipe. When measuring the cottage cheese, make sure you get even coverage with the liquid from the container.

10. swap the maple syrup for honey or brown sugar. Alternative sweeteners have not been tested.

11. you may swap the white whole wheat flour for a) ½ cup whole wheat and ½ cup all purpose flour or b) 1 cup of all purpose flour. Gluten-free, almond, oat and other alternative flours have not been tested in this recipe.

12. some cottage cheese brands are wetter than others. If your batter seems dry, add ¼ cup milk or almond milk into the batter. Compare your batter to the photos in this recipe card.

13. Storage

14. Cool pancakes completely on a wire rack before storing.

15. Fridge- stack pancakes in an air tight container and refrigerate for up to 4 days.

16. Freezer- wrap pancakes in plastic, then place in a freezer bag or meal prep container. Alternatively, stack the pancakes with squares of wax or parchment paper between them. Wrap loosely in parchment and then store in an air tight container for up to 1 month.

3. Instant Pot Breakfast Casserole

Prep Time: 15 Minutes

Cook Time: 30 Minutes

Servings: 6

Ingredients

- 6 eggs
- ½ cup milk see note 1
- 2 bell peppers finely chopped
- ½ cup frozen spinach chunks leave frozen; see note 2
- 1 cup cheese shredded; mozzarella or cheddar
- ¼ teaspoon salt
- 4 slices bacon cooled + chopped

Instructions

1. Mix together ingredients- in a bowl or large measuring cup, beat the eggs. Mix in the milk, bell peppers, frozen spinach, salt, bacon and ⅔ of the shredded cheese.

2.

    egg mixture for breakfast casserole in bowl

asserole in bowl

3. Prepare the Instant Pot- place 1 cup (for the 6 quart) or 1.5 cups (for the 8 quart) in the stainless steel insert of the Instant Pot. Place the trivet on top and a well-greased 7 inch cake pan (*note 4) on the trivet.

4. nd cake pan

5. Add egg mixture- carefully pour the egg mixture into the cake pan. Sprinkle the top with reserved shredded cheese.

6. Cover- carefully work a piece of aluminum foil over the pan, working the edges around the cake pan. It does not have to be super tight.

7. Cook- Place the lid on the Instant Pot, set the steam release handle to 'sealing', and pressure cook on high pressure for 30 minutes. Once the Instant Pot beeps, perform a quick pressure release by carefully transferring the steam release handle to the 'venting' position.

8. Tips:

9. you may swap dairy milk for unsweetened almond milk.

10. make sure you use spinach that is frozen in small pieces and not one big chunk; if your spinach comes in a block, thaw and press moisture out before mixing

it in. If using fresh spinach, sauté until softened so it mixes into the eggs properly (raw spinach will float).

11. nutritional information is for ¼ of the casserole.
12. springform pans are not great for this recipe as they leak
13. Storage
14. This recipe stores and reheats really well.
15. Fridge- Cool completely, then store the casserole in individual meal prep containers.
16. Freezer- Cool completely, then wrap individual slices in plastic wrap. Store in a larger freezer bag or meal prep container for up to 3 months.
17. Reheating
18. Thaw completely before heating. Heat in the microwave until steaming hot.

4. Gluten-Free Strawberry Streusel Muffins

Prep Time15 minutes

Cook Time25 minutes

Servings: 12

Ingredients

For the muffins:

- 2 cups blanched almond flour
- ½ cup coconut flour
- 6 eggs (preferably pasture-raised)
- ½ cup raw honey
- 1 tsp vanilla extract
- ½ tsp unrefined sea salt
- 1 cup strawberries (chopped – frozen or fresh)
- 1 tbsp butter
- 1 tsp baking powder
- coconut oil or butter (to grease muffin pan)

For the streusel:

- 3 tbsp coconut oil (softened butter)
- 4 tbsp blanched almond flour

- ¾ cup walnuts (finely chopped)
- 3 tbsp honey
- ⅛ tsp cinnamon

Instructions

1. Preheat your oven to 350 degrees Fahrenheit. Place unbleached muffin cup paper liners in a standard muffin tin. If you're not using muffin cups, grease the muffin tin with coconut oil or butter.
2. Chop strawberries into small pieces and set aside.
3. In a small bowl, mix together the streusel ingredients and set them aside.
4. In a large bowl, combine the muffin dry ingredients: almond flour, coconut flour, baking powder and salt.
5. In a medium bowl, whisk together the eggs, honey, melted butter and vanilla, then add the wet ingredients to the dry ingredients and them together. Gently fold in the strawberries with a spoon or spatula.
6. Divide the muffin batter between nine cups. Use approximately 1/3 cup batter per muffin cup.
7. If needed, pat the batter down into rounded heaps with lightly oiled hands. Next, sprinkle the streusel topping over the batter.

8. Bake the muffins for 25-30 minutes, or until an inserted toothpick comes out clean. The top should be springy yet firm when they're ready. Enjoy!

5. Pumpkin Custard Filling

Ingredients

- 1 cup coconut cream (the cream that rises to the top when you refrigerate a can of coconut milk)
- 6 tbsp maple syrup
- 4 large egg yolks
- 1 tsp vanilla extract
- 1 tsp ground cinnamon
- ½ tsp ground nutmeg
- ½ tsp ground ginger
- ¼ tsp sea salt
- ½ cup canned pumpkin

Instructions

1. Preheat the oven to 325 degrees F.
2. In a medium saucepan, whisk coconut cream and maple syrup. Simmer over medium-high heat for about 5 minutes. Remove from the heat.
3. In a small bowl, whisk the egg yolks. Now you need to temper the egg yolks before adding them to the heated coconut cream. Do this by slowly adding 1 tbsp of the hot cream/maple syrup mixture, whisking constantly.

Then add another tbsp of the hot mixture to the egg yolks, whisking constantly. Add another tbsp of the hot mixture. Add the egg mixture to the remaining hot cream, and whisk.

4. Add the vanilla, cinnamon, nutmeg, ginger, sea salt and pumpkin. Whisk until smooth. Pour over the baked crust.

5. Bake until the custard is set in the center but not stiff which is about 45 minutes to 55 minutes. Remove from the oven and refrigerate for at least 4 hours.

6. Slice into bars.

6. Pumpkin Spice Custard with Marrow Infusion

Ingredients

- 1 small pie pumpkin
- 6 pastured eggs
- ½ cup grass-fed beef bone marrow (about 2 lbs of bones)
- ¾ cups coconut milk (substitute raw milk or cream for a decadent texture - raw cream is not readily available in my area, but fortunately the marrow imparts a similar quality)
- 1 tbsp homemade pumpkin pie spice (or 2 tsp ground cinnamon, 1 tsp ground ginger, and 1/4 tsp ground cloves)
- ½ tsp unrefined sea salt
- ½ - ¾ cup maple syrup or raw honey (to taste)

Instructions

1. Preheat oven to 350 degrees.
2. Cut -pumpkin in half and scoop out seeds.

3. Place pumpkin halves cut side down in a baking dish and add 1/4 inch water. Remove from the oven when you can easily pierce the shell with a fork (about 45 minutes - 1 hour)

4. While the pumpkin is baking, bring marrow bones to a boil and let simmer for 10 minutes. When the marrow is ready, scoop the bones out with a slotted spoon and place in a bowl to drain. After they've cooled a bit use a butter knife to extract the marrow. Place it in a small bowl.

5. Spoon marrow - but not the oil that has collected at the bottom of the bowl - in with the eggs, milk/coconut milk, cinnamon, ginger, cloves, salt and honey. Puree until smooth.

6. When the pumpkin is cooked through, scoop out the flesh and add it to the egg mixture. Blend until smooth.

7. Place mixture in ramekins or a large oven-safe dish and bake at 375. Custard placed in small ramekins should be ready in about 35-45 minutes. Large casserole dishes take about 45-minutes to an hour. Watch carefully and remove when it is set in the center.

8. Serve with whipped cream if desired.

7. Resistant Starch Bacon & Ranch Potato Salad

Ingredients

- 1½ pounds red potatoes
- 1 cup sour cream
- ½ cup raw cheddar cheese
- ½ cup green onions
- 12 ounces bacon (cooked and crumbled into pieces)
- 2½ teaspoons dried parsley
- 1½ teaspoons onion powder
- 1½ teaspoons dried basil
- ¼ teaspoon garlic powder
- ¾ teaspoon sea salt (or more to taste)
- ¼ teaspoon black pepper

Instructions

1. The day before you want to serve this potato salad, place the potatoes in a pot and along with cold water that covers the potatoes by about two inches. Generously salt the water and bring to a boil. Reduce

heat to a medium simmer and allow potatoes to cook until they're tender. The amount of time will vary based on the size of the potato, but it usually takes somewhere between 20-30 minutes. When tender, remove the potatoes from the pot and place in the fridge to cool overnight.

2. The next day, cook the bacon and set aside. Stir the parsley, onion powder, basil, garlic powder, salt and pepper into the sour cream. Chop the potatoes into pieces and place in a bowl. Add 1/2 cup green onions, raw cheddar, bacon and sour cream mixture and stir until well-combined.

8. Broccoli Cheddar Breakfast Quesadillas

Prep Time: 15 Minutes

Cook Time: 15 Minutes

Servings: 7

Ingredients

- 2 teaspoons olive oil
- 1 onion diced
- 3 cups broccoli florets cut into VERY small pieces
- 4 eggs
- ¼ teaspoon salt
- ¼ teaspoon pepper
- 1 cup cheddar cheese shredded
- 4 tortillas 12"

Instructions

1. Heat a large pan over medium heat. Add the oil and the onion, and cook for 5 or so minutes, until onion is cooked through.

2. Add the broccoli and cook for 5 more minutes, until bright green and tender.

3. While cooking the veggies, beat the eggs with the salt and pepper. Add to the pan and cook, stirring frequently, for 2-3 minutes, until eggs are cooked through. Remove from heat and allow to cool slightly.

4. In a clean pan, assemble quesadillas: on half of the tortilla, add ⅔ cup of egg mixture, topped with ⅓ cup cheddar cheese. Fold the tortilla over on itself and press firmly. Cook for 2-3 minutes per side until golden and crispy.

5. Remove from heat and cool completely on a wire rack.

6. Storage

7. Cut each quesadilla in half and stack each serving. Wrap tightly in plastic wrap, then place in a large ziplock bag. Keeps in the fridge for up to 3 days and in the freezer for up to 3 months.

8. Re-heating Thaw overnight in the fridge (if frozen), or in 30 second increments in the microwave.

9. Heat in a frying pan over medium heat 3-4 minutes per side, or in a George Foreman Grill for 2-3 minutes total.

9. Easy Baked Oatmeal Muffins

Prep Time: 10 Minutes

Cook Time: 25 Minutes

Servings: 4

Ingredients

Base Recipe:

- 1 ½ cups old fashioned oats
- ½ teaspoon cinnamon
- 1 teaspoon baking powder
- 1 large egg
- ¼ cup maple syrup
- 1 cup milk

Blueberry Almond (Makes 8)

- 1 ½ cups old fashioned oats
- ½ teaspoon cinnamon
- 1 teaspoon baking powder
- 1 large egg
- ¼ cup maple syrup or honey
- 1 cup milk

- 1 cup blueberries
- ¼ cup sliced almonds

Zucchini Chocolate Chip (Makes 8)

- 1 ½ cups old fashioned oats
- ½ teaspoon cinnamon
- 1 teaspoon baking powder
- 1 large egg
- ¼ cup maple syrup or honey
- 1 cup milk any kind
- 1 cup shredded zucchini moisture squeezed out
- ¼ cup chocolate chips

Morning Glory (Makes 10)

- 1 ½ cups rolled oats
- ½ teaspoon ground cinnamon
- ¼ teaspoon ground ginger
- 1 teaspoon baking powder
- 1 large egg
- ¼ cup maple syrup or honey
- 1 cup milk
- ½ cup applesauce
- 1 carrot finely shredded (⅓ cup)

- ¼ cup chopped pecans
- ¼ cup shredded coconut
- ¼ cup raisins or dried cranberries

Superseed (Makes 8)

- 1 ½ cups old fashioned oats
- ½ teaspoon ground cinnamon
- 1 teaspoon baking powder
- 1 large egg
- ¼ cup honey
- 1 cup milk any kind
- ¼ cup chia seeds
- ¼ cup pumpkin seeds
- ¼ cup sunflower seeds
- 2 tablespoons ground flax
- ¼ cup whole almonds

Cranberry Apple (Makes 10)

- 1 ½ cups old fashioned oats
- ½ teaspoon ground cinnamon
- 1 teaspoon baking powder
- 1 large egg
- ¼ cup maple syrup or honey
- 1 cup milk any kind

- ½ cup chopped apple
- ½ cup frozen cranberries

PB & J (Makes 6-8)

- 1 ½ cups rolled oats
- 1 teaspoon baking powder
- ¼ cup maple syrup or honey
- 1 large egg
- 1 cup milk any kind
- ½ cup natural peanut butter
- 6 teaspoons jam for spooning on top

Double Chocolate Pumpkin (Makes 10-12)

- 1 ½ cups rolled oats
- 1 teaspoon baking powder
- ½ cup pumpkin puree
- 1 large egg
- ¼ cup maple syrup or honey
- 1 cup milk any kind
- ¼ cup cocoa powder
- ¼ cup mini chocolate chips

Instructions

1. Heat oven to 350°F.
2. Line a muffin tray with silicone or parchment liners, or spray generously with spray oil.
3. In a large bowl (preferably with a spout), mix together all ingredients. Spoon into the prepared muffin liners. Try to get oat mixture and liquid evenly divided between all liners.
4. Bake for 20-25 minutes, until lightly golden and no longer jiggling.
5. Cool completely before storing.
6. Tips:
7. may be called 'rolled oats' 'old fashioned oats' or 'large flake oats'. Do not use quick oats or steel cut oats.
8. the egg may be replaced with a flax egg for a vegan version.
9. maple syrup may be swapped for an equal volume of honey or brown sugar.
10. you may use any dairy or non-dairy milk including almond, oat, macadamia nut or soy milk.
11. Storage
12. store in an air tight container in the fridge for up to 4 days

13. freeze in a freezer bag (suck the air out using a straw), or wrapped in parchment paper in a meal prep container, for up to 1 month

10. Cornbread & Sausage Stuffing

Ingredients

- 1 pan prepared gluten-free cornbread (I used a mix. You can substitute regular cornbread here. Prepare the day before.)
- 1 cup walnuts, roughly chopped
- 2 tablespoons butter
- 1 tablespoon olive oil
- 12-ounce pork breakfast sausage (I used a gluten-free sausage.)
- 1 yellow onion, diced small
- 2 celery sticks, diced small
- 1 tablespoon fresh thyme leaves, removed from the stem and chopped
- 2 tablespoons fresh sage leaves, chopped
- 3 cloves garlic, minced
- 2 eggs, slightly beaten
- 1 1/2 cups chicken stock
- 1 cup fresh cranberries
- Salt and pepper, to taste

Instructions

1. Preheat your oven to 400 degrees.
2. Dice day-old cornbread into medium-sized cubes and lay out on a baking sheet.
3. Sprinkle walnuts around cornbread and bake for 20 minutes, or until cornbread starts to brown.
4. Remove from oven and let cool completely. Reduce temperature to 350 degrees.
5. In a large skillet, heat butter and olive oil together. Add sausage and, when it begins to brown, add onion and celery.
6. Cook just until onion becomes tender, about 3 minutes. Turn off heat and let mixture cool completely.
7. In a large bowl, mix cooled cornbread mixture and cooled sausage mixture with remaining ingredients. Generously season with salt and pepper.
8. Spoon cornbread mixture into a glass baking dish (I used a 9-by-9) and cover with foil.
9. Bake for 35 minutes.
10. Remove foil and bake for 25 more minutes.

11. Spiralized Veggie Thai Noodle Bowls

Prep Time: 15 Minutes

Cook Time: 15 Minutes

Servings: 5

Ingredients

- ¼ cup creamy peanut butter
- ¼ cup soy sauce
- juice of 1 lime
- 2 tablespoons brown sugar or honey
- 1 teaspoon sesame oil
- Noodle Bowls
- 6 oz whole wheat spaghetti
- 1 tablespoon olive oil
- salt & pepper
- 1 lb raw shrimp
- 1 medium zucchini
- 2 carrots
- 1.5 cups cabbage

Garnish

- Green onion
- crushed peanuts

Instructions

1. Shake together all peanut sauce ingredients and set aside (it helps to heat the peanut butter in ten second increments in the microwave first).
2. Cook spaghetti according to package directions.
3. While pasta is cooking, cook the shrimp: heat olive oil in a non-stick pan over medium heat.
4. Add the shrimp and season with salt & pepper. Cook 3-5 minutes, turning halfway, until pink and cooked through.
5. When pasta is cooked through, drain thoroughly. Combine with the vegetables and toss in the peanut sauce.
6. Top with cooked shrimp, green onions and crushed peanuts.

12. Pesto Chicken Mug Pasta

Cook Time: 10 Minutes

Total Time: 10 Minutes

Servings: 5

Ingredients

- ½ cup pasta see notes
- 1 cup water
- pinch salt
- 1.5 tablespoons pesto
- ½ cup cherry tomatoes halved
- ½ cup spinach torn
- ½ cup cooked chicken breast cubed
- 2 tablespoons parmesan cheese
- pinch red pepper flakes

Instruction

1. Place the pasta and ⅔ cup of water in a meal mug. Sprinkle with salt.
2. Place a paper towel under the mug, and heat on high (NO LID) for 5 minutes, stirring once halfway through.

3. After the 5 minutes is up, stir the pasta and add the remaining ⅓ cup of water. Heat for 2-3 more minutes (NO LID), or until pasta is cooked through.

4. Stir in the pesto until pasta is coated. Add in the tomatoes, spinach and chicken, then microwave on high for 30 seconds-1 minute (LID ON), until spinach is wilted and tomatoes are soft.

5. Stir in the cheese, sprinkle with red pepper flakes, and enjoy!

13. Turkey Sausage And Sweet Potato Lunch Bowls

Prep Time: 15 Minutes

Cook Time: 25 Minutes

Servings: 5

Ingredients

Sweet Potatoes:

- 4-5 cups sweet potato cubes 1 inch
- 1 tablespoon olive oil
- salt & pepper generous

Sausage:

- 1 lb Italian turkey sausage 500 g
- Mixed Vegetables
- 2 bell peppers cut into 1 inch pieces
- ½ red onion chopped into 1 inch pieces
- 1-2 zucchini sliced into 1 inch pieces
- 1 tablespoon olive oil
- salt & pepper

Maple Tahini Dressing

- 2 tablespoons tahini
- 2 tablespoons water or more to thin out
- 1.5 teaspoons maple syrup
- 1.5 teaspoons lemon juice
- ⅛ teaspoon salt

Instructions

Grill

1. Heat barbecue to medium-high heat (425°F).
2. Sweet Potatoes Depending on how much space you have on your grill, you may want to make these in the oven. Toss the sweet potatoes with olive oil, salt and pepper.
3. Using a vegetable grilling basket or plate, cook the sweet potatoes, stirring often, for 15-20 minutes, or until cooked through.
4. Sausage: Pierce with a knife and grill for 10-15 minutes, turning every 2-3 minutes, until cooked through.
5. Mixed veggies: Toss veggies with olive oil and salt and pepper.

6. Grill on a vegetable grilling basket or plate, stirring every 2-3 minutes, until cooked through (10 or so minutes).

Oven

1. Pre-heat oven to 425°F. Line a baking sheet with parchment and set aside.
2. Arrange sweet potato cubes on the baking sheet, and bake for 15 minutes.
3. Give them a stir and return to the oven for another 10 or so minutes, until they are easily pierced with a fork.
4. Add the vegetables and sausages to a separate sheet pan, and cook for 10-15 minutes, until cooked through.

Assembly

1. Divide the sweet potatoes, sausages and vegetables evenly between four meal prep containers.
2. Shake together all ingredients tahini dressing ingredients. Add additional water until thinned to your desired consistency.
3. Portion out tahini dressing into condiment containers, or you may drizzle over the bowls immediately.

14. Slow Cooker Creamy Potato Corn Soup (Vegan)

Prep Time: 10 Minutes

Cook Time: 8 hrs

Servings: 5

Ingredients

- 6 cups yellow fleshed potatoes cut into large chunks
- 2 cans corn 700 mL/ 22 oz total
- 2 jalapeños deseeded and sliced
- ½ teaspoon salt
- 1 teaspoon cumin
- ½ teaspoon oregano
- ½ teaspoon ground coriander
- 3 cups stock

Before Serving:

- 1 cup Almond Breeze Original
- Juice of 1 lime
- chives

Instructions

1. Place the yellow potatoes, corn, jalapeños, salt, cumin, oregano, ground coriander and stock in a large slow cooker.

2. Cook on low for 6-8 hours or on high for 4 hours.

Prior To Serving:

1. Scoop out 6 cups of potatoes and place in a large bowl. Add the Almond Breeze Original (Unsweetened) Almond Beverage, and mash until potatoes are almost smooth (still a bit chunky).

2. Return to the pot along with the lime juice.

3. Taste and add salt and extra stock (see note) if needed.

15. Sweet Borscht and yummy

Prep Time: 10 Minutes

Cook Time: 45 Minutes

Servings

Ingredients

- 1 ounce dried porcini mushrooms
- 3 tablespoons olive oil
- 2 small onions, peeled and diced
- 5 cloves garlic, minced
- 1/4 teaspoon caraway seeds
- 1 teaspoon dried dill seeds, or 1 tablespoon chopped fresh dill
- 4 medium carrots, chopped
- 2 russet potatoes (about 1 pound total), peeled and chopped
- 1 bunch red beets (about 1 1/2 pounds total), peeled and chopped
- 4 cups water
- 2 teaspoons salt
- Juice of 1/2 lemon
- 1 tablespoon brown sugar

- 1/4 cup apple cider vinegar
- 1/2 cup chopped fresh parsley leaves, beet greens, or carrot greens
- Freshly ground black pepper
- 2 teaspoons hot sauce, plus more for serving
- Sour cream, for serving

Instructions

1. Soak the mushrooms in 1 cup very hot water for 15 minutes. Drain, reserving the liquid, and chop finely. Strain the soaking liquid through a fine-mesh strainer or a coffee filter to remove any impurities and set aside.

2. Meanwhile, heat the oil in a large stock pot over medium heat until shimmering. Add the onions and sauté until translucent. Stir in the garlic, caraway seeds, and dried dill, if using. Cook, stirring, for a minute, then add the carrots, potatoes, and beets. Cook until the vegetables start to soften, about 5 minutes.

3. Add the water, salt, lemon, sugar, vinegar, and mushrooms and their soaking liquid. Stir and bring to a boil. Reduce the heat and simmer until all the

vegetables are tender, 30 to 45 minutes. Stir in the greens and simmer for a minute until they have wilted. Taste and season with more black pepper and hot sauce as needed. LUTEN FREE + VEGAN OPWHITE CHICKEN CHILI {

16. Chiken Chill

Prep Time: 25 Minutes
Cook time: 40 Minutes
Served: 3

Ingredients
For soup

- 3/4 cup raw cashews
- 1 cup hot water + more to soak cashews
- 2 tablespoons olive oil
- 1 medium onion, diced
- 4 cloves garlic, chopped
- 1 bell pepper, diced
- 2 stalks celery, diced
- 1 small jalapeno, finely chopped (optional)
- 2 teaspoons cumin
- 1 teaspoon coriander
- 1 teaspoon garlic powder
- 1 teaspoon onion powder
- 1 teaspoon oregano
- 1 teaspoon salt
- 1/2 teaspoon black pepper

- 4 cups broth
- 1 1/2 pounds boneless skinless chicken breasts or thighs or about 3 cups pre-cooked shredded chicken (for a veg option, omit chicken and substitute with extra veggies or canned beans)
- Juice of one lime
- Salt and pepper to taste

To garnish

- Cilantro
- Avocado
- Radish
- Jalapeno
- Lime
-

Instructions

1. Soak cashews. Add cashews to a heat proof bowl and cover with just boiled water. Set aside.

2. Sauté veggies and spices. In a large soup pot heat olive oil over medium heat. Once hot, add onions, garlic, bell pepper, celery, and jalapeno pepper. Sauté until onions and peppers have softened and are starting to caramelize – about 10-12 minutes. Add cumin, coriander, garlic powder, onion powder, oregano, salt, and pepper and sauté for another 1-2 minutes, until spices are aromatic.

3. Add broth and chicken breasts and bring to a simmer. Simmer for 15-20 minutes – until chicken is cooked through. Reduce heat to low. If using already cooked shredded chicken, just simmer the veggies and broth for 10-15 minutes and add the chicken in the next step.

4. Shred chicken. Carefully remove chicken from the soup to a cutting board. Allow to cool slightly. When cool enough to handle shred using two forks or cut into bite sized pieces. Return to the soup, keeping the heat on low.

5. Prepare the cashew cream. Drain and rinse the soaked cashews and add to a high-speed blender with 1 cup of

hot water. Blend on high for a minute or two, until completely smooth and no pieces of cashew remain. Add cashew cream to the soup and stir to combine. Bring back to a simmer and cook for about 5 minutes or so – to thicken slightly and bring the flavors together.

6. Season to taste with salt and pepper and the juice of one lime.

7. Serve and enjoy! Top with Cilantro, avocado, radishes, jalapeño, and extra lime wedges if desired and serve!

17. Creamy vegetable soup

Prep Time: 30 Minutes

Cook time: 55 Minutes

Served: 3

Ingredients

- ¾ cup raw cashews
- 1 ½ cups just boiled water + more to soak
- 3 tablespoons olive oil
- 1 medium yellow onion, diced
- 3 cloves garlic, chopped
- 2 stalks celery, thinly sliced
- 4 carrots, cut into rounds
- 1 teaspoon salt
- 1 teaspoon poultry seasoning
- 1 teaspoon dried oregano
- Pinch of chili flakes (optional)
- 3 tablespoons tomato paste
- 1 14.5 ounce can diced tomatoes, undrained
- 5 cups chicken broth

- 2 boneless skinless chicken breasts – about 1 – 1 ½ pounds, or about 3 cups worth of leftover cooked shredded chicken
- A few big handfuls of baby spinach
- ¼ cup parsley, chopped
- Salt and pepper to taste
-

Instructions

1. Start by soaking the cashews for the cashew cream. In a small heat proof bowl cover raw cashews with just boiled water and set aside to soak .

2. In a large soup pot heat olive oil over medium heat and add onions, carrots, celery, garlic, and salt. Sauté veggies, stirring occasionally, for about 8-10 minutes – until soft and starting to caramelize.

3. Add tomato paste, poultry seasoning, oregano, salt, and chili flakes if using. Continue to cook until tomato paste has darkened slightly – another minute or two. This step deepens the flavor of the tomato paste and spices.

4. Add broth, diced tomatoes, and chicken breasts. Bring back up to a simmer. Simmer for about 20-25 minutes

– until chicken is cooked through and veggies are tender. Reduce heat to low. If using already cooked leftover shredded chicken, just simmer the veggies and broth together and add the chicken in the next step.

5. When chicken is cooked, carefully remove from the soup to a cutting board. Shred using two forks or cut into bite sized pieces. Return the shredded chicken to the soup.

6. Prepare the cashew cream. Drain and rinse the soaked cashews and add to a high speed blender with 1 1/2 cups just boiled water. Blend on high for a minute or two, until completely smooth and no pieces of cashew remain. Add cashew cream to the soup along with parsley and stir to combine. Bring back to a simmer and cook for about 5 minutes or so – to bring the flavors together and thicken slightly.

7. Turn off the heat. Add a few big handfuls of baby spinach and stir until wilted. Season to taste with salt and pepper.

8. Serve and enjoy!

18. Cajun Chicken Pasta

Prep Time: 25 Minutes

Cook time: 40 Minutes

Served: 2

Ingredients

- 3/4 cup raw cashews
- 12 ounces gluten free pasta
- 3 tablespoons olive oil, divided
- 1 pound boneless skinless chicken breasts, cut into bite sized pieces
- 1/2 small yellow onion, finely diced
- 1/2 a large red pepper, thinly sliced
- 1/2 a large yellow or orange pepper, thinly sliced
- 3 cloves of garlic, chopped
- 2 tablespoons tomato paste
- 1 teaspoon onion powder
- 1 teaspoon garlic powder
- 1 teaspoon dried oregano
- 1 teaspoon smoked paprika
- ¼ teaspoon dried thyme
- Pinch or two of cayenne (optional)

OR

- 2 tablespoons Cajun seasoning instead of onion powder, garlic powder, oregano, paprika, and thyme
- 1 1/2 cups broth, chicken or vegetable broth both work
- 2 tablespoons nutritional yeast
- 1 1/2 teaspoons salt, plus more to taste
- 1/2 teaspoon black pepper, plus more to taste
- Parsley, to garnish (optional)

Instructions

1. Before you start cooking – in a heat proof bowl, cover raw cashews with just boiled water for at least 30 minutes, or up to an hour. If you're in a hurry you can simmer the cashews on the stove top for about 10 minutes until they are pale and plump.
2. Start a large pot of lightly salted water to boil for the pasta. When water is boiling add pasta and cook according to package instructions. Reserve about 3/4 cup cooking water. Drain and set aside.
3. In a small bowl mix together all the dried spices – onion powder, garlic powder, oregano, paprika, thyme, and cayenne (if using) until well combined.

4. Heat 2 tablespoons olive oil over medium high heat in a large skillet. When the oil is hot, add the chicken breast pieces and sprinkle with 1 teaspoon of the Cajun seasoning mix. Cook, turning each piece of chicken so it cooks on both sides, until cooked through. Remove to a plate and set aside.

5. Add the additional tablespoon of olive oil to the skillet with the diced onion, bell peppers, and chopped garlic. Sauté veggies for about 3-4 minutes – until tender. If the bottom of the skillet gets too dark add a tablespoon or two of water to release the brown bits and reduce the heat a bit.

6. Add the 2 tablespoons of tomato paste and remaining Cajun seasoning. Cook for another minute, stirring frequently, until spices are aromatic and tomato paste has darkened slightly. Remove from the heat while you make the pasta sauce.

7. Drain soaked cashews and add to the blender with broth, nutritional yeast, 1 1/2 teaspoons salt, and 1/2 teaspoon black pepper. Blend on high for at least a minute – until entirely smooth and creamy.

8. Return skillet to the stove top over medium low heat. Add cooked pasta, cooked chicken, and the cashew sauce. Stir to combine and scrape up any brown bits

from the bottom of the pan. Bring to a simmer. Allow to simmer for a minute or two, until sauce coats the pasta and chicken. As it simmers, add the reserved pasta water a bit at a time to thin the sauce until desired consistency is reached. If you need more liquid or if you didn't reserve any pasta water, you can also use chicken broth or plain water. The more liquid you add the softer and creamier the sauce will be.

9. Taste and season to taste with salt and pepper. Top with fresh parsley if desired and serve!

19. Shrimp and Avocado Salad

Prep Time: 35 Minutes

Cook time: 60 Minutes

Served: 4

Ingredients

- 1 pound cooked shrimp, tails removed and cut into thirds
- 1 large avocado, peeled and diced or sliced
- 1 cup cherry tomatoes, cut in half
- 1 cup thinly sliced cucumbers
- 1/2 cup red onion, thinly sliced
- A few big handfuls of arugula or another tender salad green
- 1/4 cup fresh lemon juice
- 1/4 cup olive oil
- 2 garlic cloves, grated or finely chopped
- 1/4 cup fresh parsley, chopped
- 1 teaspoon kosher salt
- 1/2 teaspoon fresh cracked black pepper
-

Instructions

1. Remove tails from shrimp and cut into thirds. Transfer to a large bowl or glass tupperware.

2. In a small bowl combine lemon juice, olive oil, garlic, salt, and pepper. Whisk to combine.

3. Pour about 3 tablespoons of the dressing over the cooked shrimp and toss to combine. Transfer shrimp to the refrigerator to marinate while you prep the rest of the salad ingredients.

4. Add a few big handfuls of arugula or another tender salad green to a large bowl or platter. Top with diced avocado, cherry tomatoes, thinly sliced cucumber, thinly sliced red onion.

5. Top with marinated shrimp, leaving behind any liquid from the bottom of the bowl, and toss with desired amount of dressing and parsley. Taste and add more salt and pepper as desired.

6. Serve immediately and enjoy!

20. Healthy Chicken Patties

Prep Time: 40 Minutes

Cook time: 55 Minutes

Yield: servings 4

Ingredients

For the chicken patties

- 1 1/2 pounds ground chicken
- 1 bunch green onions, white and light green parts thinly sliced, some reserved for garnish
- 1/4 cup chopped fresh parsley or 2 tablespoons dried
- 1 egg
- 2 tablespoons coconut flour
- 1 1/2 teaspoons garlic powder
- 1 1/2 teaspoons onion powder
- 1/2 teaspoon paprika
- 2 teaspoons kosher salt, or to taste
- 1/2 teaspoon black pepper
- 3 tablespoons olive oil, plus more as needed
- Green onions, parsley, and lemon wedges to garnish (optional)

For the spicy aioli

- 1/3 cup avocado oil mayo

- 1 tablespoon Whole30 compatible hot sauce

-

Instructions

1. Mix the together the patty ingredients. Add ground chicken, green onions, parsley, egg, coconut flour, garlic powder, onion powder, paprika, salt and pepper to a large bowl and mix to combine. Allow to rest for a couple of minutes so the coconut flour can absorb some of the moisture in the mixture.

2. Form into patties and cook. Form into 8 small patties using clean hands – wetting your hands can help keep them from getting sticky. Heat a large skillet over medium heat until hot. Add 3 tablespoons olive oil and tilt the pan to fully coat the bottom. When the oil is hot and shimmering cook the patties – in batches if necessary – for about 4 minutes per side (undisturbed to keep them from sticking – see notes above in blog post for more tips) until golden brown and cooked through. A splatter screen can help keep the stove top mess at a minimum.

3. Make the spicy mayo if using. Mix mayo with hot sauce until well combined.

4. Serve and enjoy! Serve patties with spicy mayo and extra green onions and herbs if desired.

21. Garlic Ginger Chicken Kabobs

Prep Time: 30 Minutes

Cook time: 1 hour 20 Minutes

Yield: 4 servings

Ingredients

For the chicken skewers

- 2 pounds boneless skinless chicken thighs, trimmed to about 1 1/3 pounds,
- 1/2 teaspoon salt
- 1/4 teaspoon black pepper
- Avocado oil for cooking
- Green onions to garnish

For the marinade

- 1/3 cup coconut aminos
- 2 tablespoons rice vinegar
- 2 tablespoons coconut sugar (or another sweetener, omit for Whole30 option)
- 3 cloves garlic, grated or finely chopped
- 1 teaspoon ginger, grated or finely chopped

- 2 tablespoons ketchup, or tomato paste (use Whole30 compatible ketchup or tomato paste for a Whole30 option)
- 1 tablespoon sesame oil
- 1/4 teaspoon white pepper, or black pepper
- 1/2 teaspoon kosher salt

Instructions

1. Mix the marinade. In a large bowl with a lid or a large glass tupperware whisk together all marinade ingredients. Set aside.
2. Prep the chicken. Cut chicken thighs into 1 inch pieces, trimming away any excess fat and cartilage. I usually start with about 2 pounds of chicken thighs which trims down to somewhere between 1 1/4 and 1 1/2 pounds – enough for 4 servings worth of chicken. If you're using boneless skinless chicken breast, you can start with approximately 1 1/4 pounds. Add chicken pieces to the container with the marinade and toss to coat. Move to the refrigerator and allow to marinate for at least 1 hour, or up to overnight, stirring a few times throughout marinating time.

3. Soak and prep the skewers. About an hour before cooking soak wooden skewers in water, so they don't burn. When ready to cook, thread chicken pieces onto skewers and season lightly with 1/2 teaspoon kosher salt and 1/4 teaspoon black pepper.

4. To cook in the oven. Preheat the oven to 400° F. Heat about 2 tablespoons oil in a large skillet (cast iron or another heavy-duty, oven safe skillet will work best) over medium heat. Sear skewers for about one minute on each side, until nicely caramelized. Work in batches, transferring the seared skewers to a plate while you cook the others. Transfer all the seared skewers back to the skillet (if they fit) or to a parchment lined baking sheet and move to the oven. Bake for 10-12 minutes, until completely cooked through. Garnish with green onions and serve.

5. To cook on the grill. Preheat the grill to medium heat. Brush the grill grates with oil and cook skewers for about 10-15 minutes, turning occasionally, until nicely charred and cooked through. Garnish with green onions and serve.

22. Kale Chicken Caesar Salad

Prep Time: 30 Minutes

Cook time: 1 hour 20 Minutes

Yield: 5

Ingredients

For kale Caesar

- 2 small bunches of kale, ribs removed and cut into bite sized pieces, about 8 cups
- 2 teaspoons olive oil
- 1/4 teaspoon salt
- Red onion, cherry tomatoes, and avocado, as desired
- Homemade Whole30 Caesar dressing, or a store bought version
- Dairy free parmesan "cheese" (optional)
- For the seasoned chicken
- 2 large boneless skinless chicken breasts
- 1/2 teaspoon garlic powder
- 1/2 teaspoon kosher salt, or to taste
- 1/4 teaspoon black pepper
- 2 tablespoons avocado oil, ghee, or olive oil for cooking the chicken

Instructions

1. Prepare the Whole30 Caesar salad dressing and set aside. If using a store bought variety, skip this step.

2. Make the kale salad. Add cut kale to a large bowl and drizzle with 2 teaspoons olive oil and 1/4 teaspoon kosher salt. Using your hands, massage kale until softened slightly – for about 30 seconds to a minute. Drizzle kale with 1/2 cup Caesar dressing and use tongs or clean hands to toss until thoroughly coated. Add more dressing if desired. Add red onion, cherry tomatoes, and avocado if using and toss again to combine. Move to the refrigerator to keep chilled while you cook the chicken.

3. Cook the chicken. Season chicken breasts evenly with garlic powder, kosher salt, and black pepper. Heat avocado oil in a large cast iron or non-stick skillet over medium heat. Once the pan is hot and oil shimmers, add chicken breasts and cook, undisturbed, for 6-7 minutes, until they are golden brown and lift easily from the pan. Turn and cook another 6-7 minutes, until cooked through. Transfer chicken to a cutting board to rest for several minutes.

4. Serve and enjoy! Divide salad between 4 bowls. Dice the cooked chicken and add to the top of the salad.

Finish with a generous sprinkle of dairy free parmesan if desired. Serve and enjoy!

23. Thai Coconut Curry Chicken Soup

Prep Time: 20 Minutes

Cook time: 55 Minutes

Yield: 4

Ingredients

- 2 tablespoons avocado oil or toasted sesame oil
- 1/2 a medium onion, thinly sliced or chopped
- 3 cloves garlic, chopped
- 1 teaspoon ginger, grated or finely chopped
- 1/4 cup red curry paste (I used Thai Kitchen)
- 1 red pepper, thinly sliced
- 2 carrots, thinly sliced
- 1 medium zucchini, halved lengthwise and thinly sliced
- 4 cups chicken broth
- 1 13.5 ounce can full fat coconut milk
- 3 tablespoons coconut aminos
- 1 pound chicken breast, cut into bites sized pieces
- 2 cups broccoli florets
- 1 teaspoon salt, or to taste
- Juice from 1 lime

- Cilantro or basil, red or green onion, chili oil, chopped cashews, extra lime wedges to garnish

Instructions

1. Cook aromatics. In a large soup pot heat oil over medium heat. When oil is hot add thinly sliced onion, garlic, and ginger. Cook for about 2 minutes – until onions start to soften and garlic and ginger are aromatic. Add curry paste and cook for 1 minute more, stirring frequently.
2. Sauté veggies. Add bell pepper, carrots, and zucchini and stir to coat with the curry paste. Cook, stirring occasionally, for about 3-4 minutes, until veggies have softened slightly.
3. Add chicken broth, coconut milk, and coconut aminos. Increase the heat to medium high and bring to a simmer.
4. Cook chicken and broccoli. Add chicken breast and broccoli florets and continue to simmer until chicken is cooked through and broccoli is bright green and tender – about 5-6 minutes.
5. Season to taste with salt and juice of one lime. I used more than 1 teaspoon, but I also started with low sodium chicken broth.

6. Garnish and serve! Serve topped with fresh herbs, red or green onion, chili oil, chopped cashews, and extra lime.

24. Sheet Pan Shredded Chicken Tacos

Prep Time: 25 Minutes

Cook time: 55 Minutes

Yield: 3 servings

Ingredients

For shredded chicken:

- 1 1/2 pounds boneless skinless chicken thighs
- 2 tablespoons orange juice
- juice of 1 lime – about 1 tablespoon
- 2 tablespoons taco seasoning
- 1 teaspoon paprika
- 1 teaspoon garlic powder
- 1/2 teaspoon cumin
- 1/2 teaspoon dried oregano
- 1 teaspoon salt
- 1/4 teaspoon black pepper
- 1 tablespoon honey or maple syrup
- 2 tablespoons olive oil
- Juice of half a lime

For serving, as desired

- tortillas – I used grain free cassava flour tortillas
- guacamole
- shredded romaine
- pickled red onions
- cilantro
- dairy free sour cream
- sliced jalapeño

Instructions

1. Place chicken thighs in a large Tupperware or Ziploc bag. Add taco seasoning, paprika, cumin, oregano, kosher salt, black pepper, honey, lime juice, orange juice, and olive oil. Use tongs or clean hands to turn and coat chicken evenly with the marinade. Move to the refrigerator and allow to marinate for at least 30 minutes, or up to overnight.

2. Preheat oven to 425 degrees.

3. Line a broil safe baking sheet with parchment paper or a silicone mat if desired for easy clean up. Add chicken thighs to the lined baking sheet, leaving any excess marinade behind.

4. Move to the oven and bake for about 15 minutes – until completely cooked through. Remove from the

oven and transfer chicken thighs to a large cutting board. Preheat the broiler. Use two forks to roughly shred the chicken.

5. Transfer shredded chicken back onto the baking sheet and toss with any accumulated juices. Spread out in an even layer. Place the baking sheet under the broiler and broil chicken for about 3-5 minutes – until nicely browned with lots of caramelized bits. *A note on broiling: If you've lined your baking sheet with parchment paper keep a close eye on your sheet pan during broiling, as parchment paper can start to burn under the intense heat. Alternatively, if you prefer your chicken to be more saucy / juicy you can skip the broiling step all together and serve the chicken immediately after shredding.

6. Remove from the oven and season with the juice of 1/2 a lime. Assemble the tacos with any desired toppings and DIG IN!

25. Buffalo Cauliflower

Prep Time: 30 Minutes

Cook time: 50 Minutes

Yield: 3 servings

Ingredients

- 1 large head of cauliflower, about 2 1/2 – 3 pounds – cut into florets, about 5–6 cups worth
- 3 tablespoons avocado oil
- 1/4 teaspoon garlic powder
- 1/4 teaspoon onion powder
- 1/2 teaspoon salt
- 1/4 teaspoon fresh cracked black pepper
- 1/2 cup buffalo sauce
- To serve: vegan ranch dressing and cut celery sticks (optional)

Instructions

1. Preheat oven and prep ingredients. Line a baking sheet with parchment paper and preheat oven to 425 degrees Fahrenheit. Cut cauliflower and gather and measure ingredients.

2. Roast cauliflower. Add cauliflower to a large bowl and toss to coat with avocado oil, garlic powder, onion powder, kosher salt, and black pepper. Transfer to a large baking sheet and spread out flat side down in a single layer. Reserve the bowl for the next step. Roast for 15-17 minutes – until just barely tender and starting to brown.

3. Toss with buffalo sauce. Remove cauliflower from the oven and increase the heat to 475°. Transfer cauliflower florets back to the large bowl and pour buffalo sauce over the top. Toss gently to coat, and transfer back to the baking sheet, leaving any excess sauce behind.

4. Roast again. Transfer back to the oven and continue to roast for an additional 6-8 minutes, until nicely caramelized on the edges. For extra crispy bits you can broil for 1-2 minutes before pulling from the oven – just keep an eye on it so the cauliflower and/or parchment don't burn.

5. Serve and enjoy! Remove from the oven and lightly drizzle with any remaining buffalo sauce from the bowl. Serve with vegan ranch dressing and celery sticks if desired and enjoy!

26. Quesadillas

Prep Time: 20 Minutes

Cook time: 55 Minutes

Yield: 2 servings

Ingredients

- 12 6-inch (15-cm) whole wheat tortillas
- 1–2 cups (120–240 grams) of Monterey jack cheese, shredded
- 15-ounce (425-gram) can of black beans, drained
- 1 onion, diced
- 1 green pepper, diced
- 1 teaspoon (1.5 grams) of garlic powder
- 1 teaspoon (6 grams) of salt
- 1 teaspoon (2 grams) of ground cumin
- 1/4 teaspoon (1/4 gram) of dried oregano
- 1/2 teaspoon (1 gram) of chili powder
- olive oil cooking spray

Instructions

1. Preheat the oven to 420°F (216°C).

2. Spread the tortillas on a lined sheet pan, ensuring it's fully covered. The tortillas should hang a bit over the edge of the pan, as they will be folded up.

3. Top the tortillas with cheese, black beans, green peppers, chopped onions, and spices.

4. Fold the tortillas over the fillings and add 2–3 more tortillas to cover the center.

5. Spray the quesadilla with cooking oil and place another sheet pan on top.

6. Bake for 20–25 minutes. Then, remove the top sheet pan and bake for an additional 10–15 minutes or until crisp and slightly golden.

7. Remove from the oven, slice into squares, and add toppings of choice.

27. Eggplant Parmesan

Prep Time: 30 Minutes

Cook time: 45 Minutes

Yield: 3

Ingredients

- 1 large eggplant, cut into thick slices
- 2 eggs
- 1 cup (119 grams) of breadcrumbs
- 2 cups (475 mL) of marinara sauce
- 1/3 cup (30 grams) of Parmesan cheese, grated
- 1 tablespoon (4.5 grams) of Italian seasoning
- 1 teaspoon (1.5 grams) of garlic powder
- 1–2 cups (225–450 grams) of mozzarella cheese, shredded
- 1/3 cup (6 grams) of fresh basil

Instructions

1. Preheat the oven to 450°F (232°C).
2. Lay sliced eggplant in a single layer on a paper towel and sprinkle with salt on both sides. Let sit for 10–15 minutes, then pat dry.

3. Whisk the eggs in a small bowl and set aside.

4. In a separate bowl, mix breadcrumbs with garlic powder, Parmesan cheese, and Italian seasoning.

5. Dunk each slice of eggplant into the egg mixture. Then, cover in the breadcrumb mixture and place in a single layer on a lined baking sheet.

6. Bake for 30 minutes, flipping halfway through.

7. Remove the sheet pan from the oven and top each eggplant slice with marinara sauce and mozzarella cheese.

8. Bake for an additional 15–20 minutes, top with fresh basil, and serve.

28. Stuffed Sweet Potatoes

Prep Time: 30 Minutes

Cook time: 45 Minutes

Yield: 3 servings

Ingredients

- 4 large sweet potatoes (about 2 pounds total), scrubbed and patted dry
- 2 tablespoons olive oil
- 1 small yellow or white onion, finely chopped
- 1/2 teaspoon salt
- 1 (15-ounce) can black beans, drained and rinsed
- 1/4 cup water
- 1 finely chopped canned chipotle in adobo chile
- 1 tablespoon plus 2 teaspoons sauce from can of chipotles in adobo, divided
- 1 medium lime, halved, divided
- 1/2 cup whole-milk plain Greek yogurt
- 1 medium avocado, diced
- 2 tablespoons chopped fresh cilantro leaves and tender stems

Instructions

1. Arrange a rack in the middle of the oven and heat to 425°F. Line a rimmed baking sheet with aluminum foil. Prick each sweet potato in four or five spots with a fork. Place them on the baking sheet and bake until very tender, about 1 hour. Meanwhile, make the chipotle black beans.

2. Heat the olive oil in a large skillet over medium heat until shimmering. Add the onion and cook, stirring occasionally, until softened and translucent, 3 to 5 minutes. Stir in the salt.

3. Add the beans, water, chipotle chile, and 1 tablespoon of the adobo sauce. Cover and reduce the heat to maintain a simmer. Cook for 5 minutes. If there's any remaining water in the pan, simmer the mixture uncovered until evaporated. Remove from the heat, squeeze in the juice of half the lime, and stir to combine.

4. Make the chipotle yogurt by stirring the Greek yogurt and remaining 2 teaspoons adobo sauce together in a small bowl.

5. Once the sweet potatoes are cool enough to handle, cut them in half lengthwise, leaving the bottom intact. Create a pouch for the filling by gently pushing the

ends of the sweet potato toward each other. Divide the black bean filling over the sweet potatoes. Top with diced avocado, chipotle yogurt, and chopped cilantro. Squeeze the remaining half of the lime over the sweet potatoes and serve.

29. Thai Chicken Buddha Bowlsi Chicken Buddha Bowls

Prep Time: 20 Minutes

Cook time: 50 Minutes

Yield: 2 servings

Ingredients

- 1 cup farro
- 1/4 cup chicken stock
- 1 1/2 tablespoons sambal oelek (ground fresh chile paste)
- 1 tablespoon brown sugar
- 1 tablespoon freshly squeezed lime juice
- 1 pound boneless, skinless chicken breast, cut into 1-inch chunks
- 1 tablespoon cornstarch
- 1 tablespoon fish sauce
- 1 tablespoon olive oil
- 2 cloves garlic, minced
- 1 shallot, minced
- 1 tablespoon freshly grated ginger
- Kosher salt and freshly ground black pepper, to taste

- 2 cups shredded kale

- 1 1/2 cups shredded purple cabbage

- 1 cup bean sprouts

- 2 carrots, peeled and grated

- 1/2 cup fresh cilantro leaves

- 1/4 cup roasted peanuts

For The Spicy Peanut Sauce

- 3 tablespoons creamy peanut butter

- 2 tablespoons freshly squeezed lime juice

- 1 tablespoon reduced sodium soy sauce

- 2 teaspoons dark brown sugar

- 2 teaspoons sambal oelek (ground fresh chile paste)

Instructions

1. To make the spicy peanut sauce, whisk together peanut butter, lime juice, soy sauce, brown sugar, sambal oelek and 2-3 tablespoons water in a small bowl; set aside.
2. Cook farro according to package instructions; set aside.
3. In a small bowl, whisk together chicken stock, sambal oelek, brown sugar and lime juice; set aside.
4. In a large bowl, combine chicken, cornstarch and fish sauce, tossing to coat and letting the chicken absorb the cornstarch.
5. Heat olive oil in a large skillet over medium heat. Add chicken and cook until golden, about 3-5 minutes. Add garlic, shallot and ginger, and cook, stirring frequently, until fragrant, about 2 minutes. Stir in the chicken stock mixture until slightly thickened, about 1 minute; season with salt and pepper, to taste.
6. Divide farro into bowls. Top with chicken, kale, cabbage, bean sprouts, carrots, cilantro and peanuts.
7. Serve with spicy peanut sauce.

30. Broccoli Frittata

Prep Time: 30 Minutes

Cook time: 55 Minutes

Yield: 2 servings

Ingredient

- 6 ounces cooked chicken breast diced or shredded
- 1 tablespoon extra virgin olive oil
- 2 cups broccoli florets chopped
- 1 large red bell pepper or orange, diced
- 3 green onions chopped
- 2 cloves garlic minced
- 1/2 teaspoon kosher salt
- 1/4 teaspoon black pepper
- 8 large eggs
- 1/2 cup sharp cheddar cheese freshly grated

Instructions

1. Place rack in the center of your oven and preheat oven to 350 degrees F. Lightly coat a 9-inch pie dish with cooking spray.

2. If your chicken is not yet cooked: Cook and shred chicken.

3. Heat the olive oil in a large skillet over medium heat. Add the broccoli and peppers and sauté until they are beginning to soften, about 5 minutes. Add the green onions, garlic, salt, and pepper and cook 1 additional minute. Remove from heat and set aside.

4. In a large bowl, whisk together the eggs, then add cheese, chicken, and the vegetables from the skillet. Stir to combine, then pour into the prepared pie dish.

5. Bake 40 minutes, until the center is nearly set and a toothpick inserted comes out clean. Remove and let sit 5 minutes then serve warm or at room temperature. The frittata will puff while baking, then settle a bit as it cools.